I0844207

McAnderson Patrick

1

FOREVER YOUNGER

SIMPLE SKILLS THAT MAKE YOU LOOK 20 YEARS YOUNGER THAN YOUR ACTUAL AGE

TABLE OF CONTENT

Calves liver

Whitefish

Picked herrings

Olive oil

Pens, beans, lentils, and vegetables

Water

Cocoa

Green tea

Soup

Cashews

Oats, quinoa, pearl grain

Kiwi natural product

Pomegranates

Citrus natural products

Salmon

Keep away from super handled food

Chapter Three

Drink coffee or tea

Eat a ton of strong plant food sources

Make an effort not to glut

Assess turmeric

Eat more nuts

Chapter Four

Conclusion

INTRODUCTION

Aging is a natural process that comes upon every living being as time passes by. As we age, our skin continue to develop wrinkles and we also loss the beautiful shape that everyone including ourselves admired while we were young. Though aging is a natural process that cannot be stopped completely, aging can at least be slowed down through the kind of foods we consume and of course the kind of lifestyle we live.

McAnderson is a nutrition expert and has offered countless services that yields fruitful results to his customers. McAnderson does not only offer nutritional services but also offer advices based on the kind of lifestyle to live so as to look at least 20 years younger than your actual age. McAnderson also recommends the types of foods to consume with their respective quantities in order to live a longer and healthier life.

CHAPTER ONE

Utilize these for your morning meal

From very good quality serums and strips to creams, it seems like there are vast items out there to accomplish more youthful-looking skin. In any case, here's a sensation that could get a good deal on skincare: what you eat can significantly affect how your appearance looks. Maturing is inescapable, yet research has shown that a significant number of the nutrients, minerals, and different substances in your food sources might assist with dialing back the interaction a piece. Furthermore, why not start your day by giving your skin a lift? Various breakfast food sources make you look youthful, all loaded with those skin-upgrading supplements.

Maturing is a characteristic interaction and nothing to be embarrassed about, Nonetheless, there are sure food sources that can assist us with dealing with the skin we have surprisingly well.

Breakfast Frankfurter

There are a few natural justifications for why your skin's appearance changes as you age. For one's purposes, your body produces 1% less collagen consistently after you turn 20 — and collagen assumes a critical part in holding your skin back from hanging. By your 40s, your skin isn't delivering any more collagen, and as it loses flexibility, kinks and barely recognizable differences start to shape all the more quickly. In the meantime, openness to UV beams and free extremists in the climate can make considerably more harm to the skin.

Wearing sunscreen consistently, abstaining from smoking, and restricting your time in the sun are all actions you can require to safeguard your skin from harm. In any case, as per the American Institute of Dermatology, eating an even eating routine with a lot of new leafy foods may likewise help avert untimely maturing, while an eating routine that is weighty in sugar and refined starches can speed up maturing.

In light of that, the following are a modest bunch of hostile to maturing food sources you ought to add to your morning meal plate

1.   Egg

Whether you lean toward them mixed, broiled, or hard-bubbled, specialists concur that eggs are an astounding decision for breakfast with regards to supporting your skin. this is simply because egg has both vitamin D and protein content.Vitamin D can safeguard skin against UVB harm, As we age, our body's capacity to create vitamin D decays, so it is critical to devour it through food varieties. Protein is additionally significant and the individuals who consume abstains from food low in protein have been displayed to have more noticeable appearance of kinks.To against maturing make an omelet with veggies like spinach, kale, or chime pepper to get a portion of L-ascorbic acid to assist with lighting up the skin's appearance.

These decisions likewise contain Vitamin E and K which will assist with advancing bloodstream, can decrease the presence of dim spots on the skin, and saturate the skin.

2. Natural product smoothie

Now is the right time to start up that blender first thing because, organic product smoothies are loaded with cancer prevention agents that can avoid harm to the skin from free revolutionaries.

Another effective method for keeping the skin hydrated is the smoothies, this has plenty advantages when it comes to improving skin. You may also add butter, hemp seeds, peanuts and avocado to smoothies for more kick of omega unsaturated fats and Vitamin E to advance skin wellbeing and lessen the irritation.

3.   Avocado

Uplifting news assuming you love to have avocado toast for breakfast: smooth green natural product is an amazing wellspring of monounsaturated unsaturated fats, which studies have shown can assist with safeguarding the skin from untimely maturing.

Omega 3 unsaturated fats, which are found in avocados, can likewise assist with further developing skin dryness, keeping skin hydrated is key in permitting it to be solid as we age.

4.   Blueberries

Christensen proposes beating your morning bowl of oats or yogurt with blueberries which are overflowing with polyphenols, which have known defensive impacts that forestall early indications of skin maturing.

Research has uncovered that polyphenols can go about as a sunscreen, assisting with shielding your skin cells against harm from the UV beams the sort that prompts wrinkles.

5. Chia seed pudding

Discussing omega-3s, chia seeds are crammed with them. That is one justification for why making a chia seed pudding for breakfast is suggested. Omega-3 unsaturated fats help to diminish aggravation, yet in addition assist the skin with keeping up with dampness which is significant for keeping it looking full and young.

 consuming more omega-3 unsaturated fats can assist with whiting platelets to safeguard small portions of DNA called telomeres, which are referred to as abbreviate over the long run as a result of maturing. Omega-3 supplementation was additionally found to decrease oxidative pressure brought about by free extremists.

6.   Tofu scramble

On the off chance that you're a vegetarian, trade the egg scramble for a delicious tofu one. Tofu contains protein, which is one of the structure squares of skin cells, as well as soy isoflavones, which have been found to lessen wrinkles and further develop skin flexibility essentially.

Tofu is a decent wellspring of zinc, which assists with forestalling free extreme harm in the body and helps in cell fix. Therefore tofu can be of great value to your skin and even every cell within your body. Include veggies and some avocado along with everything else and you've additionally got extraordinary wellsprings of cell reinforcements and phytonutrients to safeguard the skin.

7. Yams

You should trade those customary hashbrowns or home fries for yams — they contain carotenoids, strong cell reinforcements got from vitamin A that have photoprotective characteristics, and the importance they'll safeguard your skin from harm. They're likewise loaded with L-ascorbic acid, which has a significant impact on skin recovery. Studies have shown that ladies beyond 45 years old who had a lower admission of this nutrient were bound to have wrinkles.

A relationship has been seen between low L-ascorbic acid admission and having dry skin, which can prompt expanded wrinkling, L-ascorbic acid insufficiency can likewise affect collagen combination, which is significant for skin versatility

8.   Tomato

At the point when the skin is presented to light the skin's lycopene can be annihilated, Food varieties like tomatoes contain lycopene, which might moderate harm. Take a stab at including salsa on top of your eggs or add cuts to avocado toast.

Studies have shown that lycopene, the phytochemical that makes this vegetable red, makes a calming difference and diminishes your skin's aversion to UV radiation. Tomatoes are likewise plentiful in B nutrients, which have hostile to maturing properties and may decrease sun harm, age spots, barely recognizable differences, and kinks while additionally adding to cell fix.

CHAPTER TWO

Extraordinary food varieties that give you more youthful looks

It's not unexpected said excellence comes from the inside and that incorporates what you eat. While there are no marvel food sources to return to some time in the past, you can look and feel more youthful by reliably eating a sound, supplementing the stuffed diet. Here are some top age-sealing food sources to day to day in corporate.

Almonds

A recent report showed that almonds diminished wrinkle appearance and pigmentation in fair-looking, postmenopausal ladies who consumed a little more than two everyday small bunches of the nuts for almost a half year. The review was incompletely supported by California Almonds, however, did freely to elevated requirements. Almonds are wealthy in skin-accommodating fundamental unsaturated fats, as well as providing almost 7mg of cancer prevention agent vitamin E - all that anyone could need to meet your day-to-day needs - per 28g modest bunch.

Carrots

Carrots and other orange-red products of the soil - like tomatoes, red peppers, yam, melon, and apricots - cosmetically affect (Caucasian) skin, upgrading its brilliant shine. They're all wealthy in carotenoids a kind of normally happening color. A concentrate in the diary Social Biology tracked down this expanded individuals' view of facial engaging quality.

Raspberries, strawberries, blueberries

Delectable berries are chockful of anthocyanins - powerful cell reinforcement and mitigating fixings that safeguard against collagen breakdown. Also, anthocyanins seem to help the strength of stomach microscopic organisms, which thusly can decrease age-related bone misfortune.

Calves' liver

Copper adds to typical hair pigmentation and examination has shown a connection between lower levels and the early appearance of white hairs. The best copper sources are sheep's and calves' liver, as well as nuts and seeds (Brazils, cashews, sunflower seeds) and crabmeat.

Whitefish

Haddock, cod, or some other white fish is loaded with iodine, a supplement the UK populace is inadequate in (we rank seventh among the ten most iodine-lacking nations internationally). Iodine isn't simply crucial to keep your digestion started up, yet it keeps skin sound as well.

Picked herrings

Another off-putting fixing that has an expected enemy of maturing benefits, cured herring, also known as rollmops, is incredibly high in vitamin D. That is great for future-sealing your skeleton, yet there could be a likely advantage for fighting off the presence of silver hairs as well. In one little review, untimely turning gray was related to lower levels of vitamin D, iron, and calcium.

Olive oil

In a review including Swedes, Greeks, and Australians, those with a higher admission of monounsaturated fat, especially olive oil, had less wrinkling in a sun-uncovered site (the rear of the hand) than the people who leaned toward spread and margarine. Vegetables and heartbeats were additionally connected with less wrinkling.

Peas, beans, lentils, and vegetables

One hypothesis concerning why beats (vegetables) could help safeguard against skin harm and kinks is their substance of normal plant estrogens (phytoestrogens). There's proof to propose that these can assist with further developing the water content of the skin, as well as shield skin cells from oxidative pressure.

Water (a lot of it)

It merits rehashing: drinking a lot of water is great for your tone. In one review, young ladies who were requested to drink an additional 2 liters of water a day saw expansions in hydration that were sufficient to "emphatically sway typical skin physiology". In excellence talk that is plumped out, smoother skin.

Cocoa

An evening cup of cocoa can be a marvel supporter - simply pick one with high happiness of flavanol cancer prevention agents, which are the key fixing that loosens up veins. The research proposes one cup of high-flavanol cocoa, for example, Aduna Super Cacao or FlavaMix ex-pat nds blood and oxygen stream to the skin and diminishes sun-related burn risk.

Green tea

Drinking a couple of day-to-day cups has additionally been connected with less skin harm. Any kind of tea is great, yet have a go at changing to green tea for the most elevated level of a key cell reinforcement known as epigallocatechingallate (ECGC). Cell culture concentrates on it's been displayed to safeguard against contamination related to skin maturing.

Soup

A major bowl of vegetable soup is an incredible method for guaranteeing you get your 5-a-day and feed your skin, hair, and nails with the supplements they need. A Dutch report observed a measurably critical relationship between soup eating and fewer kinks in senior ladies.

Cashews

Cashews have over two times the iron convergence of barbecued lean ribeye, which might assist with checking balding, keep you ruddy-cheeked and fight off incapacitating weakness. They are additionally a decent wellspring of zinc, which can help in mending skin breakouts.

Oats, quinoa, pearl grain

These are the lower glycaemic record (more slow delivering) sugars that you ought to be attempting to get into your eating regimen (as opposed to the higher GI ones like potatoes, rice, and white bread). A lower glycaemic record diet brings down your gamble of spots, while higher glucose levels are related to looking more established.

Kiwi natural product

A terrible night's rest can add a long time to your face. A recent report in the diary Rest observed that individuals appraised sleepless people as having more kinks/scarce differences and droopier mouths. For a superior opportunity for a peaceful evening, eat two or three melatonin-containing kiwi natural products before bed. In a little clinical preliminary restless people revealed better rest quality and daytime working after eating the natural product before bed.

Pomegranates

Pomegranates and pomegranate juice are overflowing with phytochemicals (a sort of compound found in plants) that add to better maturing, generally because of calming impacts. A human pilot investigation discovered that a compound called urolithin in pomegranates eased back muscle misfortune and improved mitochondrial work (the capacity of cells to deliver energy), which could convert into looking and feeling more youthful for longer.

Citrus natural products

An everyday aid of citrus will ensure you'll get sufficient L-ascorbic acid, which has been connected with less creased and dry-looking skin. One orange supplies over two times the base suggested admission. Other incredible wellsprings of L-ascorbic acid are peppers, nectarines, strawberries, and salad greens.

Salmon

A rich and delicious wellspring of omega-3 fats, salmon is the vital element of the Perricone weight reduction diet that indicates to causes the skin to show up more energetic. Omega-3s are calming, and have likewise been accounted for to safeguard against UV harm. There's a decent equilibrium between protein and veggies in the Perricone diet so on the off chance that you're hoping to launch feeling better for the most part, as well as care for your skin, this 72-hour plan is a reasonable method for making it happen. Continuously address your PCP before beginning any eating routine.

Keep away from super handled food

Sweet, greasy accommodation food with flavorings, emulsifiers, and different added substances considered as "super handled" (we're checking out at your treats, sausages, exquisite tidbits, and moment noodles). Keep away from an excessive amount of super-handled food on the off chance that you need to live longer, as a high admission has been connected to more limited telomere length. Telomeres are the grouping of hereditary material at each finish of your chromosomes. More or less, more limited telomere lengths imply you are maturing quicker.

CHAPTER THREE

Food sources that advance life span

1. Drink coffee or tea

Both coffee and tea are associated with a lessened bet of diligent ailment. For instance, the polyphenols and catechins found in green tea could lessen your bet of a dangerous development, diabetes, and coronary disease. Coffee is associated with a lower opportunity of type 2 diabetes, coronary ailment, and certain harmful developments and frontal cortex affliction both coffee and tea shoppers benefit from a 25-35% lower risk of early passing appeared differently about non-purchasers Essentially remember that an unnecessary measure of caffeine can similarly incite strain and lack of sleep, so you could have to take a look at your admission to the proposed farthest reaches of 400 mg every day around 4 cups of coffee. It's furthermore vital that it overall requires six hours for caffeine's assets to subside. As such, expecting you to experience trouble getting adequate incredible rest, you could have to move your admission to earlier in the day. Moderate usage of tea and coffee could help sound development and life expectancy.

2. Eat a ton of strong plant food sources

Gobbling up a wide combination of plant food assortments, similar to natural items, vegetables, nuts, seeds, whole grains, and beans, may reduce disease endanger and propel life range. For example, numerous examinations associate a plant-rich eating routine with a lower peril of abrupt passing, as well as a diminished bet of threatening development, metabolic confusion, coronary sickness, demoralization, and psyche rot. These effects are attributed to laying out food sources' enhancements and cell fortifications, which integrate polyphenols, carotenoids, folate, and L-ascorbic corrosive

As requirements are, a couple of assessments interface veggie darling and vegan thins down, which are ordinarily higher in plant food sources, to a 12-15% lower chance of unforeseen passing. Comparative assessments similarly report a 30-55% lower risk of kicking the pail from harmful development or heart, kidney, or compound-related contaminations. Similarly, some assessment suggests that the bet of abrupt passing and certain infections increases with more unmistakable meat usage. Regardless, various examinations report either nonexistent or much more delicate associations — with the unfavorable results seeming, by all accounts, to be unequivocally associated with taking care of the meat. Veggie darlings and vegans in like manner all around will frequently be more prosperity perceptive than meat-eaters, which could be mostly to sort out these revelations.

By and large, eating a ton of plant food assortments is most likely going to assist prosperity and existence with traversing. Eating a great deal of plant food assortments is likely going to help you live longer and lower your bet of various typical ailments.

3. Make an effort not to glut

The association between calorie confirmation and life expectancy right currently delivers a lot of interest. Animal examinations recommend that a 12-53% abatement in conventional calorie confirmation could increase the best future

Examinations of human masses popular for life length similarly notice joins between low-calorie utilization, a somewhat long future, and a lower likelihood of infection What's more, calorie limit could help with decreasing overflow of body weight and girth fat, the two of which are connected with more restricted futures. Taking everything into account, long stretch calorie impediment is regularly unfeasible and can consolidate negative delayed consequences, such as extended hunger, low inner intensity level, and a decreased sex drive. Whether calorie impediment moves back develops or grows your future isn't yet totally appreciated.

4. Assess turmeric

Concerning threatening developing philosophies, turmeric is an unimaginable decision. That is because this flavor contains an extraordinary bioactive compound called curcumin.

In light of its cell support and moderating properties, curcumin is made sure to help with staying aware of the brain, heart, and lung work, as well as defend against harmful developments and age-related contaminations. Curcumin is associated with an extended future in the two bugs and mice. In any case, these disclosures have not always been imitated, and no human examinations are at present open. Before long, turmeric has been consumed for centuries in India and is, all things considered, seen as safeguarded.

5. Eat more nuts

Nuts are feeding powerhouses. They're rich in protein, fiber, cell fortifications, and worthwhile plant compounds. Likewise, they're an unimaginable wellspring of a couple of supplements and minerals, similar to copper, magnesium, potassium, folate, niacin, and supplements B6 and E A couple of assessments show that nuts beneficially influence coronary sickness, hypertension, disturbance, diabetes, metabolic turmoil, belly fat levels, and, shockingly, a couple of kinds of infection. One examination found that people who consumed something like 3 servings of nuts every week had a 39% lower chance of unforeseen passing. Additionally, two late studies including more than 300,000 people saw that individuals who ate nuts had a 5-29% lower chance of passing on during the audit period — with the best abatements found in the people who ate 1 serving of nuts every day. A couple of nuts to your regular timetable could keep you sound and help you with living longer.

CHAPTER FOUR

CONCLUSION

Now that you have gone through the book with carefulness, it is very important to make sure you apply all the knowledge acquired in this book. To gain knowledge without application is as good as useless. Apply the simple techniques in this book in order to fulfill your dreams of looking younger than your actual age and as well as living a longer and healthier life.